Survivor Tales

SALLY JO MARTINE

DEDICATION

"Survivor Tales" is dedicated to my sister, Shirli Barovich, whose compassion, tireless support, and practical assistance made my journey with breast cancer bearable.

It's also a tribute to my mother, Helen Martin, whose courage and fortitude inspired my own.

AUTHOR'S NOTE

These handmade, one-of-a-kind original monkeys discovered themselves somewhere between the assemblage of their body parts and subsequent adornment.

Each monkey has their own story, yet they share a common purpose – to bring levity, light, and joy into the lives of others.

VISIT US ONLINE

OneBeingHuman-sjm.com

ACKNOWLEDGMENTS

After receiving my breast cancer diagnosis, the sock monkey journey expanded from playful to political to grieving and meaning-making. Despite countless twists and turns, the monkeys' lighthearted ways kept the whole project on track. Along the route, the monkeys encountered numerous fans whose presence and support supplied me with the courage and strength to keep moving forward. Specifically, I'm grateful to my mother, Helen Martin and my aunt, Val Richardson for capably demonstrating "happy living after breast cancer." Dr. Linda Pai and Dr. Todd Willcox delivered impeccable surgical expertise with a kindness and confidence into which I could relax. Dominique Cantwell and the entire Bainbridge Performing Arts' staff and board remained steadfast in their support of both my recovery and my pursuits with primates. Alan Francescutti captured each monkey with the stealthy skill of a wildlife photographer, and Don Flora generously supplied design guidance. This book benefited immeasurably thanks to last-minute scrutiny and inventive suggestions from Alex and Don. I can't imagine where I or the monkeys would be without my primary primate fans. You know who you are! I want to extend a huge thank you to the Bremerton Friends of the Library– your enthusiasm is infectious. And sincerest gratitude to the Puget Sound Affiliate of Susan G. Komen® for its dedication to combating breast cancer on every front. All photographs are courtesy of Alan Francescutti unless otherwise noted.

A NOTE ABOUT GENDER

While it is true that all of the characters depicted in this book are female, it is not my intent to ignore the incidence of breast cancer in males. The American Cancer Society reports that approximately 1% of all breast carcinomas occur in men, and many of them die from it. My exclusive focus on females merely reflects my own sense of relative authority.

BANDIT

Bandit spent years thinking of her breast cancer "detour" as stealing the best years of her life. She thought of those days as a sort of side trip that didn't really have anything at all to do with her real journey. They formed a remote counterpart to the healthy, safe story that her life really was. Now, however, being faced with the cancer's return, she began to wonder if there was something important here, something that actually had everything to do with who she was, how she was, and what she was going to do with the time she had. Maybe this wasn't just something to be "gotten through;" maybe it was central to her being alive. By dismissing a part, was she endangering the whole? If she sat openly enough, could she find room to hold both joy and pain? By embracing all of herself, could she recover her sense of wholeness?

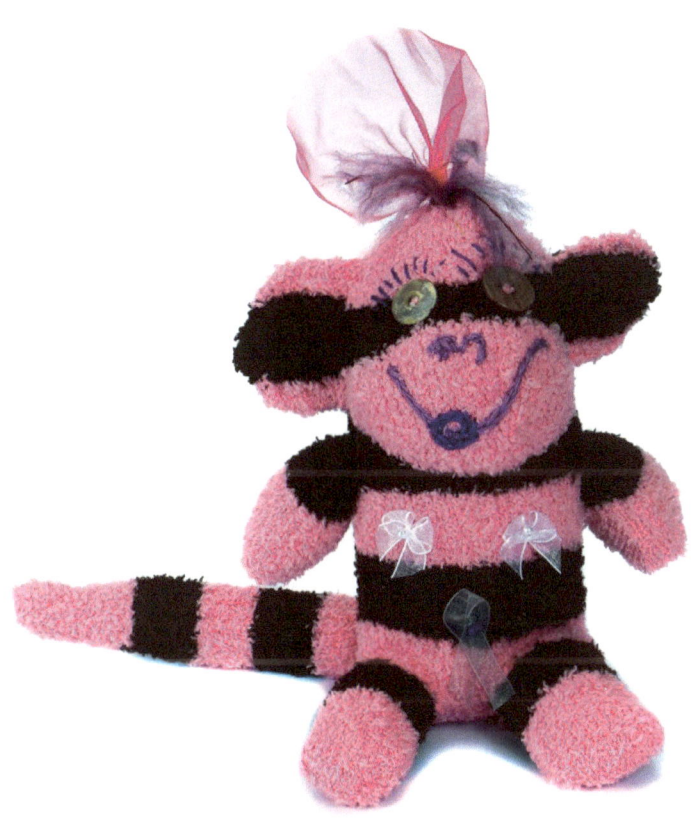

BETTE

Bette's eyes pooled up and she rapidly blinked back her tears. Though the doctors said she was now cancer-free, and all of the experts said she could resume unrestricted activity, she still felt the loss, and it swamped her sometimes. The emotional ache wasn't something she carried front and center, but it crept up unannounced. Like the other day when she heard about a new technique for dealing with phantom limb pain. An ingenious and surprisingly inexpensive solution for those with missing arms and legs, it sadly wasn't a viable method for addressing the physical pain she often felt in her missing breasts. She was glad for the promise "mirror therapy" held for amputees, but the grief of her own loss welled up as she heard the story. She was thankful to have room to grieve when the need surfaced, but she was equally relieved to know that things were always in motion, and that although the pain was fierce, it wasn't everything.

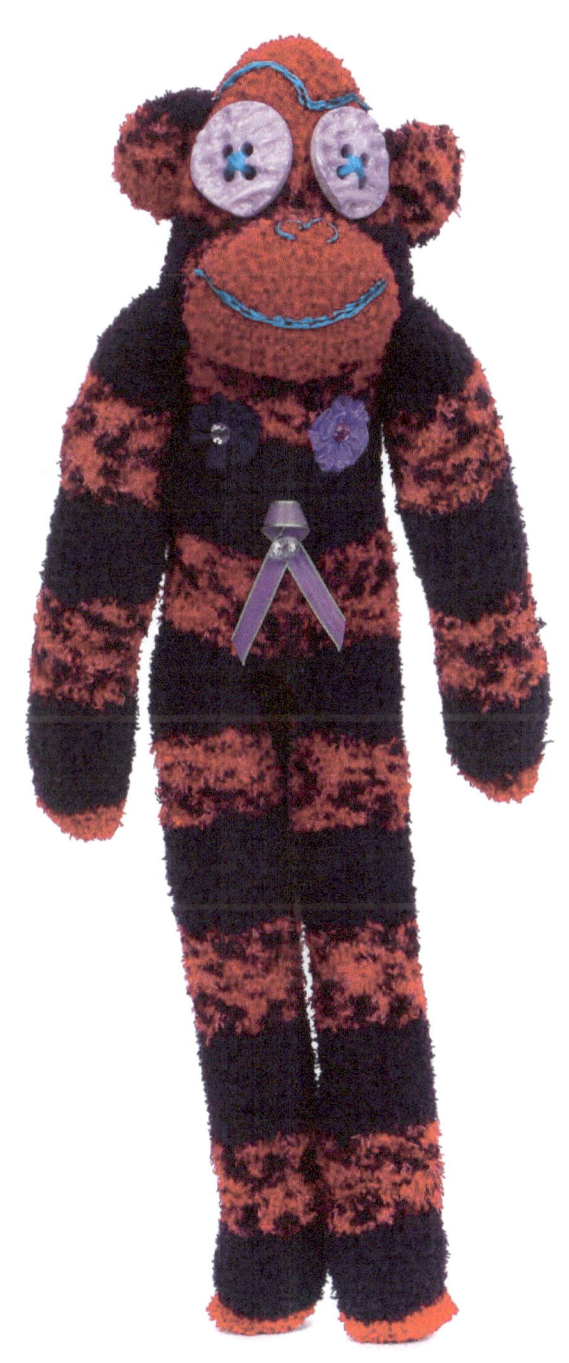

BONITA

True to her name, Bonita was lovely, and she had a wide open heart, which she shared freely with everyone she met. The trouble with an open heart flame was that it attracted both lovers and moths. In other words, she was just as vulnerable to pain and loss as she was sensitive to joy and abundance. Accordingly, she was carefully discerning. Filtering was a way of life. She didn't want the people and ideas she entertained to become a steady stream of noise. Her pose of openness required a delicate balance – remaining open while observing boundaries mandated the focus of a warrior. While expansive, she knew her heart reserves and energy were finite, so she amortized her energies across a field of choice. When she received her diagnosis, she set it down. She sat with it. She looked at it. And she tenderly reflected on how she was going to interact with it.

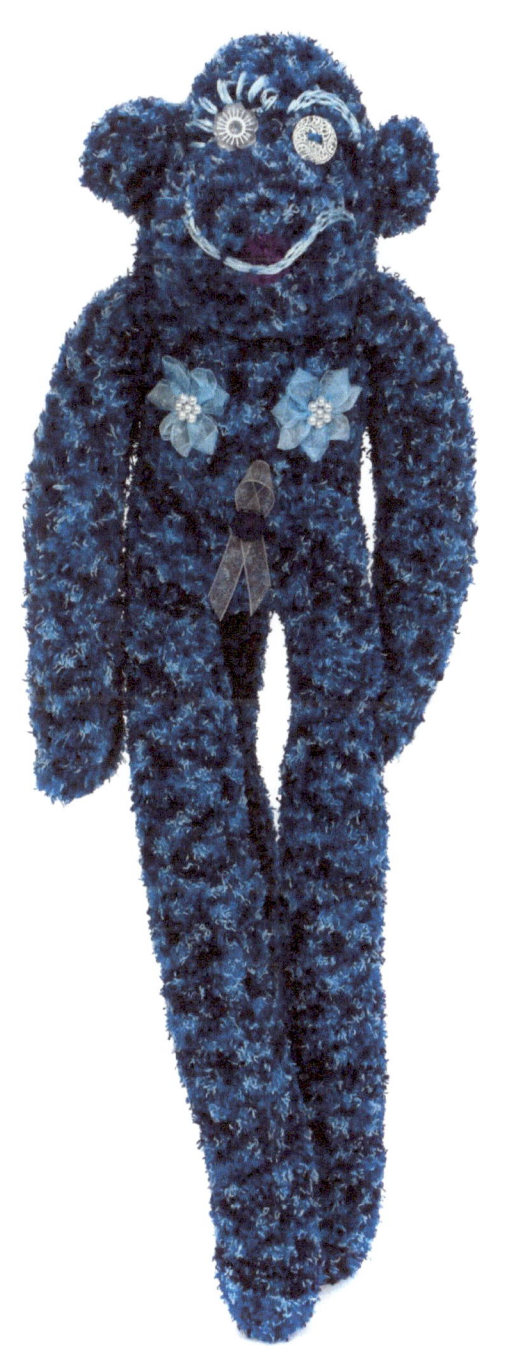

BRENDA

The diagnosis certainly did throw a wrench in Brenda's plans. She was booked up from here to the next millennium. She had micromanaged her dance card to the extent that every second seemed consumed...swallowed up in a frenzy of activity that left her mind buzzing. Now she had to squeeze in doctors' appointments and lab tests. Ridiculous! She would have to clone herself. That's what she needed to do. She sniggered. Now that was absurd – cloning would merely replicate the terminal gene, and she would still wind up dead. She stared long and hard at her to-do list. What was on it that was so damn critical? If she wasn't here to do it, none of it was going to get done anyway. And "taking care of herself" wasn't even on the list. What did that say about her priorities for goodness sake? She saw that she was going to need to do some serious chiseling to that to-do list right now. Resistance wasn't going to help matters. Somehow, she had to find the courage to get out of her own way.

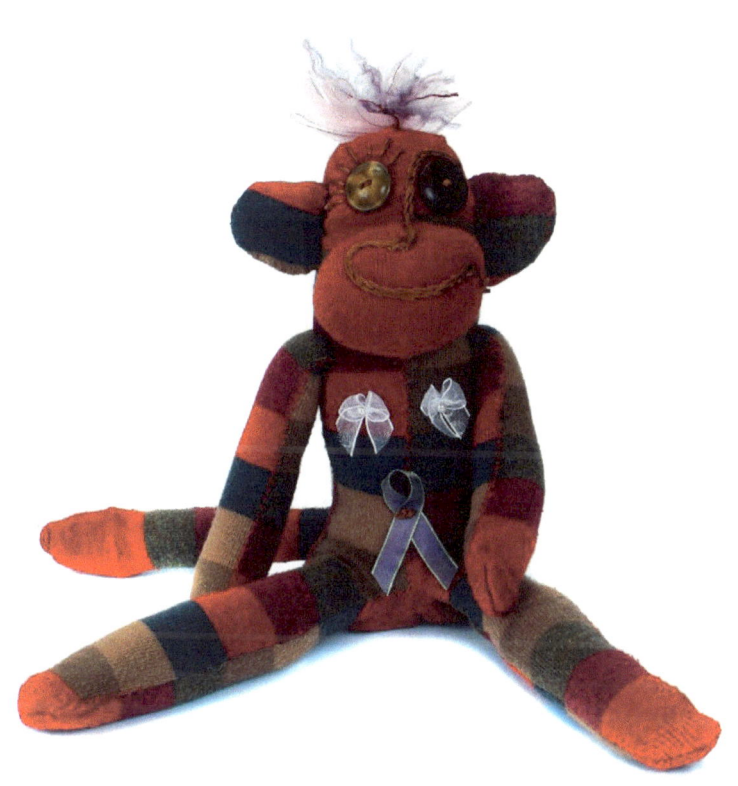

FAITH

Faith was thriving on all fronts when news of an abnormal mammogram came in. In one fell swoop, life as she "planned" it sputtered and ground to a halt. Dazed and bewildered, she watched helplessly as her sense of control slipped away. Long priding herself as a strong and independent monkey, Faith is slowly acquiring the necessary courage to seek out and receive help from others. What's emerging is a meaningful journey that is reshaping her world from the inside out. She is now bringing a resilient voice to the local breast cancer community where she works to promote interdependence with her fellow monkeys. Photo courtesy of Rex-zane Rudee, Hudson Photography.

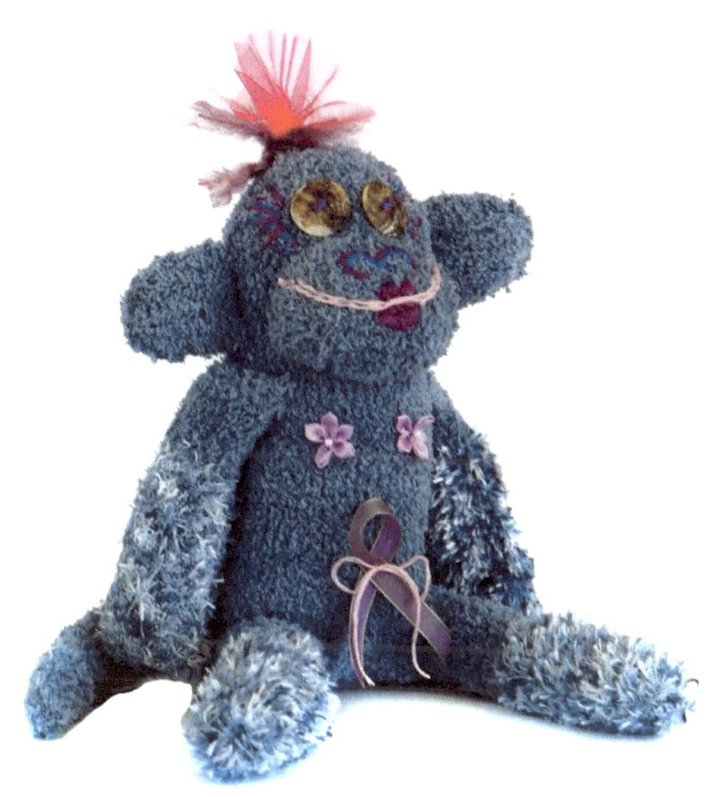

GAIETY

Coming from a long line of schoolmarms, Gaiety learned early in life about the importance of taking things in stride. Her grandmother was the wizened matriarch of her clan, and she dispensed wisdom with a firm tone and unyielding stance, adhering rigidly to established norms of right and wrong. In this strict environment, Gaiety readily absorbed the tribally-tested posture of fitting in and blending seamlessly. She suspected there was value to be gained from a more flexible stance, but she was a pragmatic sort, and she kept that awareness to herself. She knew her grandmother loved her, despite her seemingly harsh ways, and she was thankful now for the strength her grandmother instilled. It was the firm ground of her upbringing, the social grooming of her tribe, and her own adaptable attitude that kept Gaiety's spirit resilient as she underwent radiation, chemo, and IV therapy.

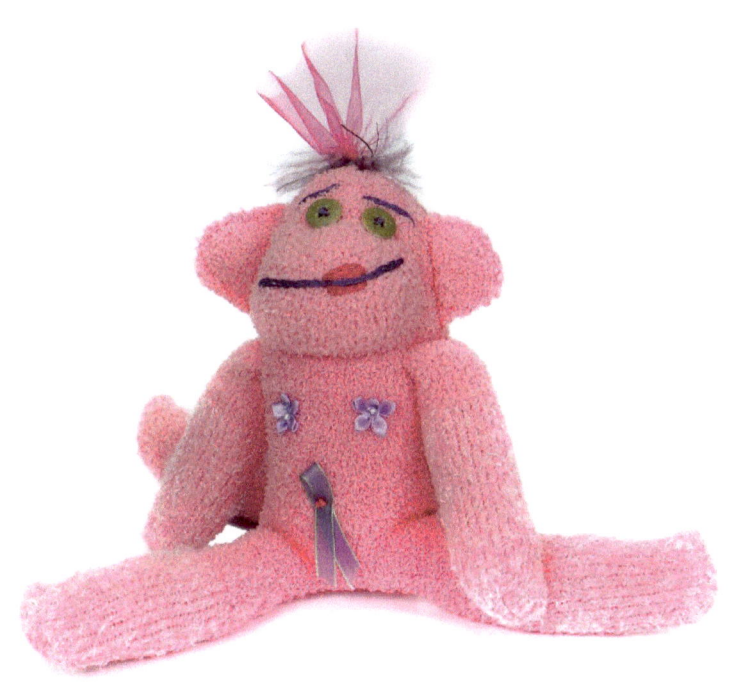

GIGI

A fun-loving monkey with a luscious figure, Gigi began attracting suitors as soon as she hit puberty. Her perfectly-formed breasts earned the envy of females and became the focus of desire for males near and far. As smart as she was beautiful, she soon hinged her entire identity on beauty and brains. It was from this vantage that she later received her diagnosis of breast cancer, and her identity rapidly collapsed, falling in a shambles at her feet. Having elected reconstruction, she underwent a weekly series of injections following her mastectomies, and she was mortified by the lack of identification she felt with her new breasts. To top things off, her typically above-average intellect was severely impaired by the pain meds. In the wreckage of her known world, Gigi began sifting through the shards. Out of this quiet, gentle activity, she noticed aspects of her identity that had previously lain dormant, and, slowly... carefully... she began piecing together her heart.

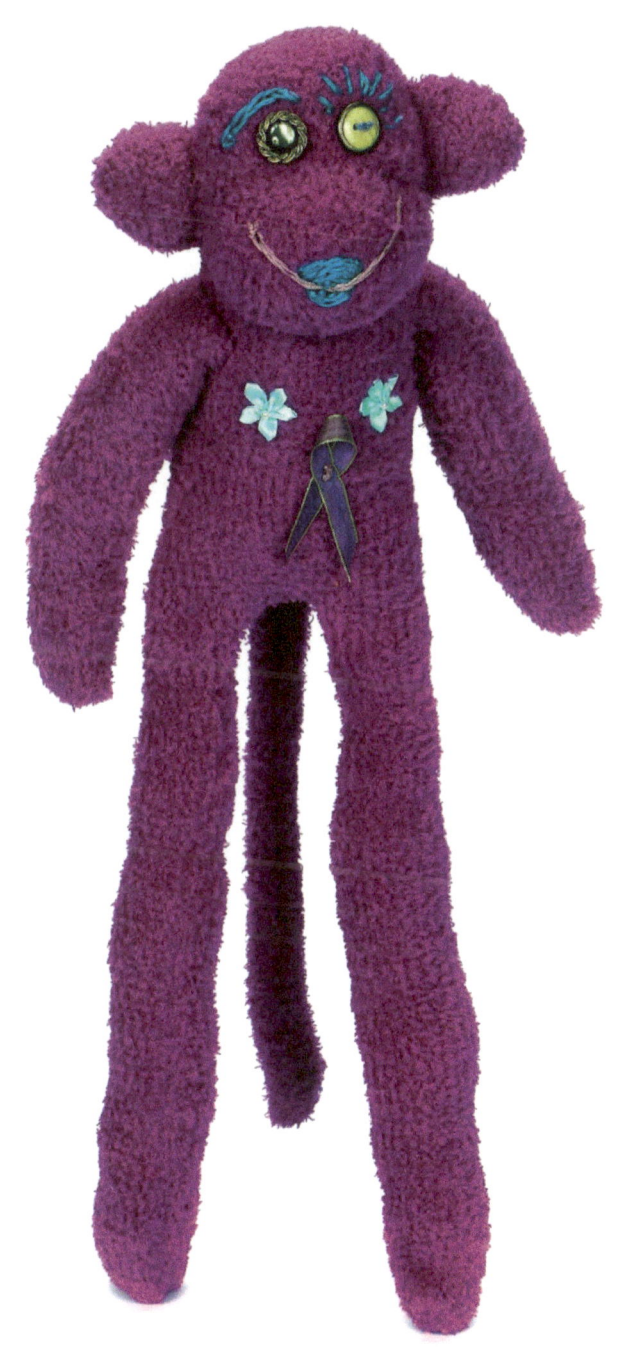

JOY

Joy came completely undone when news of her cancer came in. It knocked her off center and sent her into a full tilt. Her ever-ready smile had shaped her countenance since she was a little girl. Her whole life was an expression of "joy." But recently she felt the smile faltering. She was hard pressed to contain the conflicting feelings at war within her. Thankfully, the training central to her upbringing had revolved around acceptance. Her parents always said, "By embracing your challenges, you'll uncover the buried treasure of their many joys." Their instruction was proving useful as she struggled to remain upright against the onslaught of turbulent feelings and physical trials.

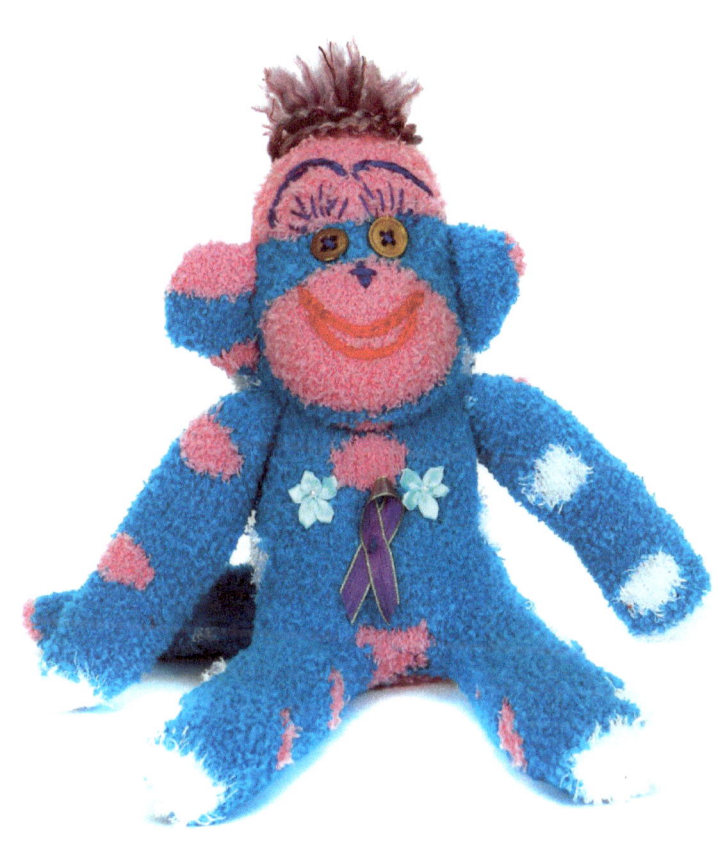

LOBELIA

Bolstered by her new membership in a virtual community of survivors, Lobelia found herself regaining interest and a sense of purpose, moving away from her role of passive bystander and toward that of active participant. A staunch opponent of positivity for positivity sake, Lobelia found herself admittedly comforted by the persistently upbeat tones of her new circle of friends. Normally, their incessant chirping would be an absolute turn off, but given how far she had fallen, she found herself clutching handfuls of hope wherever and whenever she could. She was pleased to note that the sky was not falling. Yes, there were some clouds overhead and storms rimming the horizon, but she could still see bits of the blue sky, and it was still up there, while she was here...grounded.

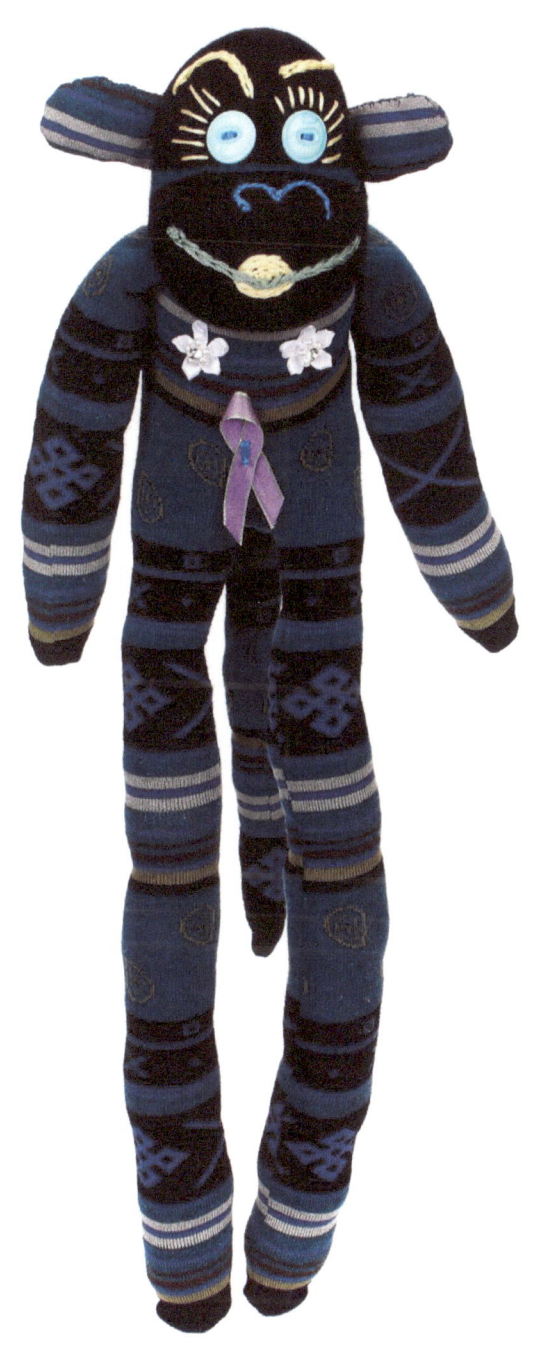

LUCY

Walking and weight lifting were, in large part, what Lucy lived for. Or, at least, they're what facilitated her life. Collaboratively they supported her physical and mental health in ways that nothing else did. Lucy often achieved a meditative state when walking. Her treks paved an opening through which the endorphins poured in, relieving the anxieties collected in the course of each day. Weight lifting served an equally vital role, making her feel strong, capable, and independent. Since the surgery, however, her activities were specifically restricted for a period of months, and both her mind and body were in revolt. She knew she "should" feel fortunate to have her life, even if she wasn't presently able to live it according to her preferences. It was tricky though, because her physical activities were central to her core identity, and her sense of self felt threatened. The coping skills on which she routinely drew were unavailable, precisely at a time when she needed them most. She was jittery, and she impatiently counted the days. She knew one thing for certain: she would participate in the annual Komen Puget Sound Race for the Cure!

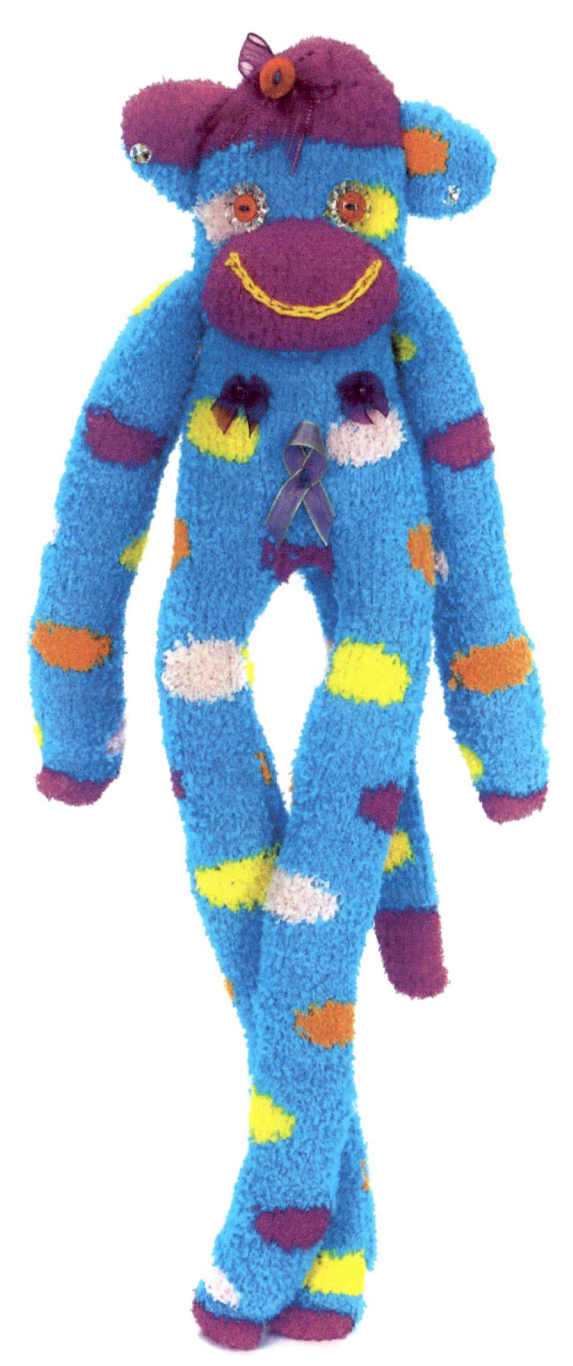

LUELLA

Luella sighed in disgust. She had just dodged the second robocall from the not-for-profit hospital billing department in as many weeks. She was presently in remission, but the physical, emotional, and financial toll of her recovery was severe. Luella was saddled with thousands of dollars of out-of-pocket health care costs above and beyond her annual deductibles. She was fortunate to have a job, a meager income, and insurance, yet she still had to apply for financial assistance. She was denied because the hospital counted her small retirement fund from a previous job as "income," this despite the distressing ramifications of accessing the account. It seemed just plain wrong to live in a society without universal health care coverage! What on earth did monkeys do who lacked even a basic health plan? Financial worries were hardly conducive to healing, and Luella was determined to advocate for the cause once her energy was restored.

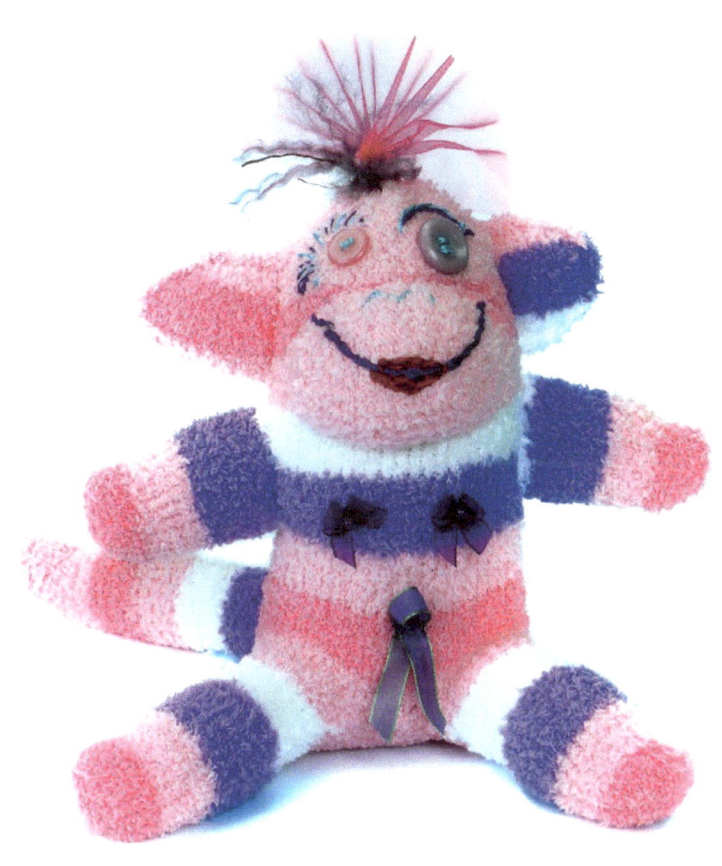

MAGGIE

Alarmed by the questions that came up during the pre-admission interview, Maggie was bereft after leaving the doctor's office. "Who was going to drive her to the hospital?" And, "who was going to be there with her for the first 48 hours following her release from the hospital?" Her parents were deceased, her siblings estranged, and as an introvert in previously terrific health, she hadn't placed "making friends who will help in an emergency" at the top of her to-do list. Yet here she was in just such an emergency. She knew she was one of those quiet types the media harped on about relentlessly, and, given her reclusive tendencies, her neighbors probably regarded her with suspicion. Whereas most monkeys sought the hive-like activity of a tribe, Maggie preferred solitude, spending hours each day reading, writing, and philosophizing about the meaning of life. The simple mechanics of her diagnosis and early treatment options were daunting, and she was surely going to have to stretch beyond her comfort zone. To whom could she turn for help? She certainly couldn't afford to pay someone. She needed to find out what resources were available through the local cancer-support organization and go from there.

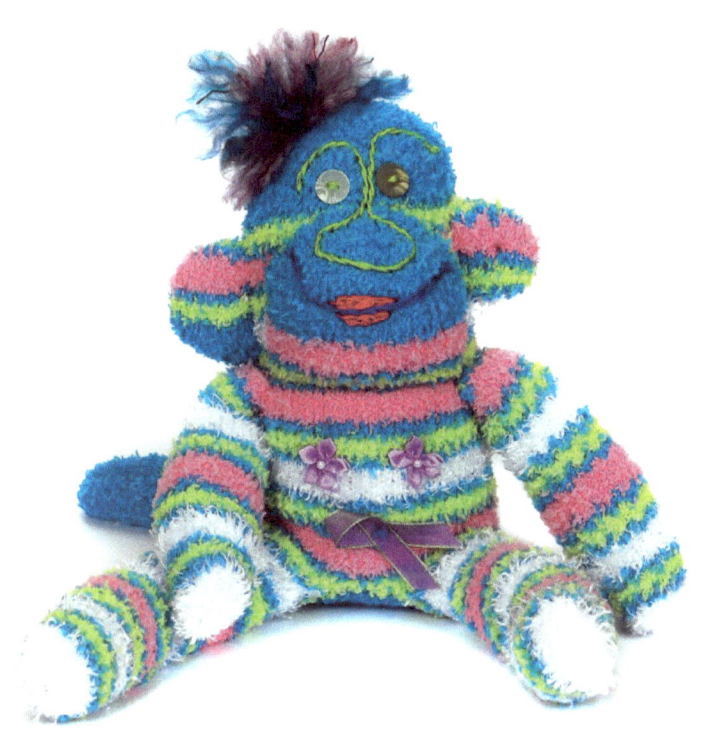

MANGO

Mango was a self-assured young monkey and a high-powered executive. She routinely out-witted her competitors and was renowned in the industry for her decisive action and confidence. Scrutinizing every conceivable move in advance, she would sweep in with incisive, intricate deals before challenges (or challengers) solidified. When news of her cancer diagnosis breached the office walls, Mango's friends and enemies anticipated swift, detached action followed by a rapid return to business as usual. But Mango's foundation had been shaken to the core, and she found herself second-guessing her every move. Retreating from the limelight, she pondered the breadth and depth of her uncertainty and became immobilized by the full weight of her unknowing. Aside from faith, speculation, inference, or theory, how could she really "know" anything? Maybe certainty wasn't all it was cracked up to be. She thought she would simply try trusting her instincts, putting one foot in front of the other, and making the most of each moment.

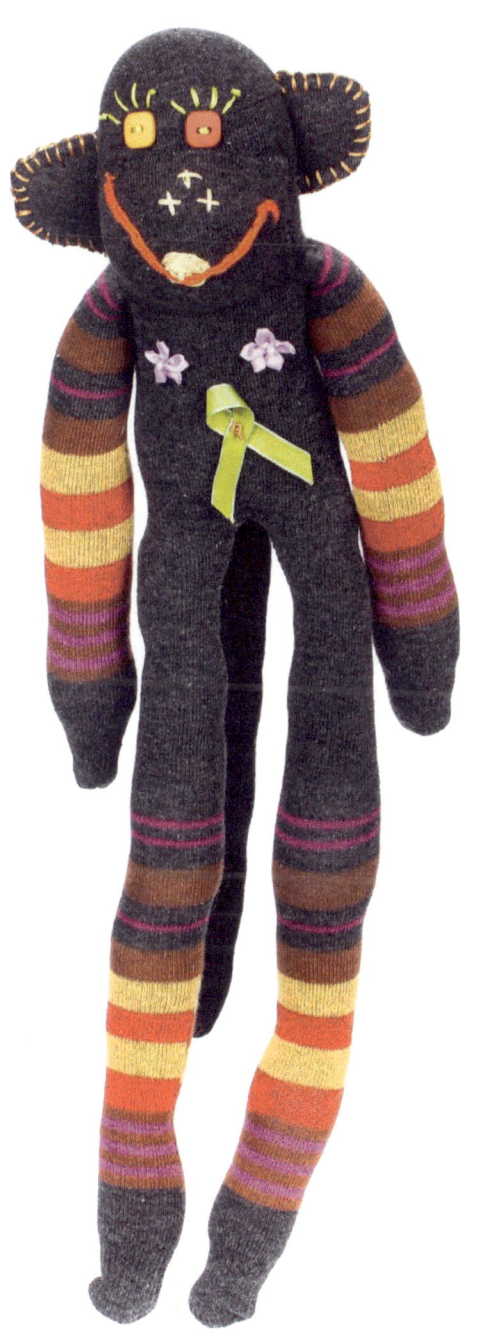

MARTHA

Diagnosed fairly late in life, Martha had made it nearly 20 years with only one breast, and she hadn't regretted her single-mastectomy decision yet. She never considered reconstruction and didn't even invest in a prosthetic. She refused to put stock in the idea that a female's breasts were a critically defining aspect of her beauty. In fact, Martha found the very idea offensive. The attitude was merely one more male-dominated means of commodifying women, and the evidence of women's ongoing objectification was everywhere. Even the tooth paste commercials these days seemed to require a flash of cleavage. A bra-burner of the 60's, Martha was frustrated living in a world that reduced everything to eye candy, sound bites, and short-term gratification. There were life-threatening issues to get riled up over, and as far as she was concerned, her cancer-induced, one-breast shortage hardly deserved her emotional energy. She had rallies to attend, causes to support, and candidates to back.

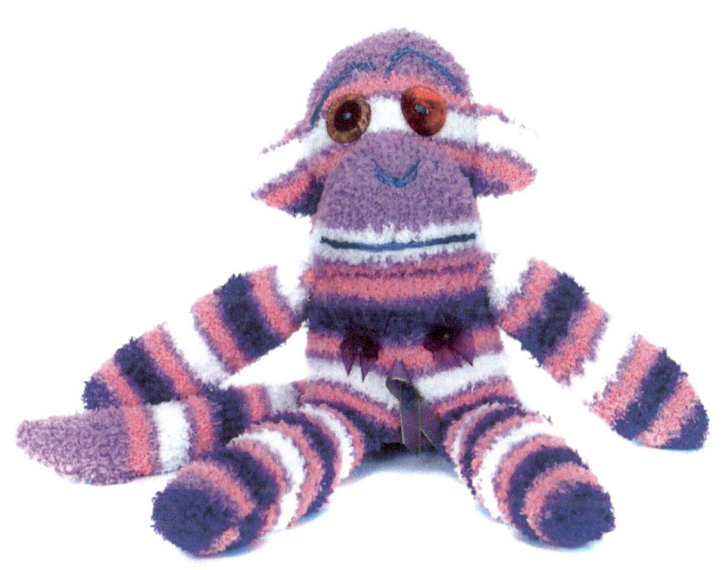

MARYANN

Ever since her diagnosis, Maryann had undergone a relentless stream of appointments. Wave after wave of consults, surgeries, and lab work pitched against her foundation, rocking her to the core. Probed and prodded, she was routinely stripped down to her body stocking, inciting the shame of exposure again and again. Though lithe and lovely in her middle years, Maryann was intensely body conscious during her pre-teens, and each new medical visit stirred up the awkward embarrassment and inhibitions that plagued her youth. The mere act of having a body was somehow shameful in the prudish sphere of her family, and her early breast development deepened her sense of humiliation. Her budding sexuality intensified her inner angst, and her identity became intimately linked to her breasts as they grew to symbolize both shame and fertility. Now that her breasts were gone, she was morphing yet again. In tandem with her ongoing physical reconstruction, she began mending her fragile identity fragment by friable fragment. She was acutely aware of the intricate ways in which her personal journey was shaped by the prevailing cultural idealization and idolization of the female form.

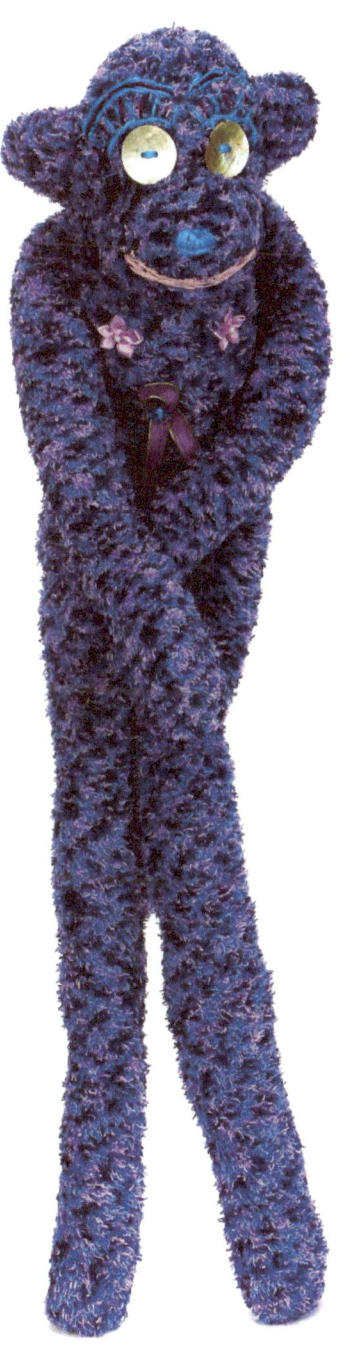

MATILDA

The world closed in on Matilda as soon as she heard him use the term "cancer." The doctor's mouth opened and closed as though he was trying to tell her something, and his expression suggested it was something important. But Matilda simply stopped hearing. Her ears closed right up, and her entire focus narrowed. "Will I be one of the survivors?" She had endured so much already, and it seemed inconceivable and unfair that she was being called to yet another test. She knew there were others with fates far worse than hers. Famine, genocide, and poverty were rampant across the globe. Even in her own community, people had lost their jobs, and many were homeless, and in the town next over, survivors were grappling with the latest school shooting. Still... hadn't she personally endured enough? Hadn't she paid her dues with the premature loss of her mate and her child? Where did she acquire this idea that life was fair?

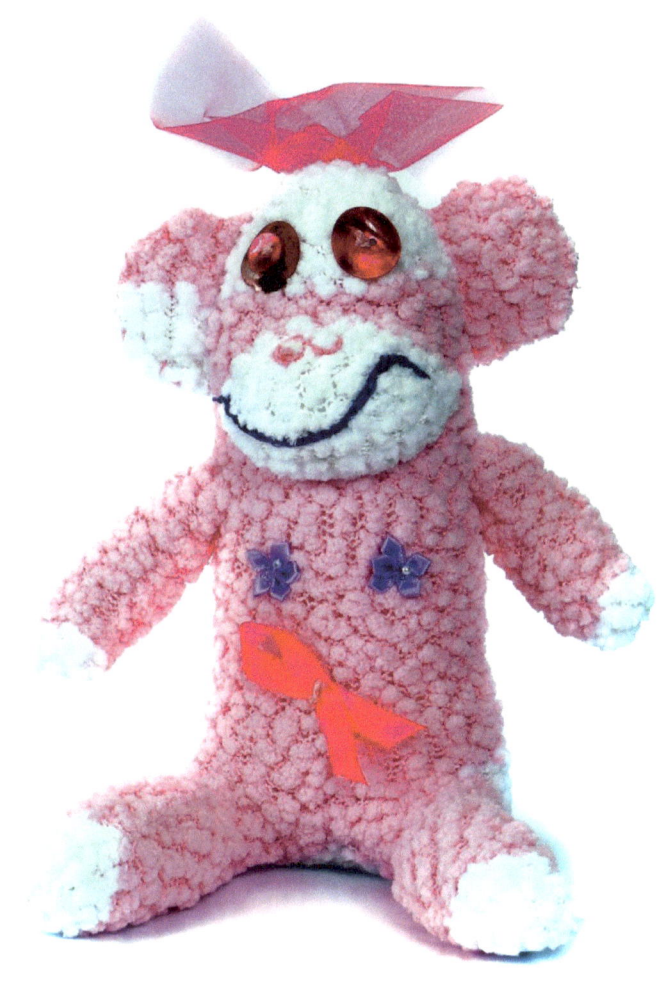

MOLLY

Her 40th year had been an extra hard one for Molly. Her boyfriend put the brakes on, her mother had passed away, and now this – the x-ray showed a lump! She would have been entirely adrift if not for her sister's anchoring support. Despite her many losses, she considered herself fortunate. Her sister made herself entirely available to her. She was there to drive her, accompany her, amuse her, and console her, waiting patiently for Molly's adjustment at each turn of the road. How many people didn't have someone to hold their hands on such a perilous journey? Her sister's kindnesses were individually small but plentiful, and collectively they served to keep Molly upright. She didn't think she could have made it without her unwavering support, and she knew now that if she made it through this, she was going to have to find some way to give back to her breast cancer compatriots – those who lacked the loving support that she was so blessed to have.

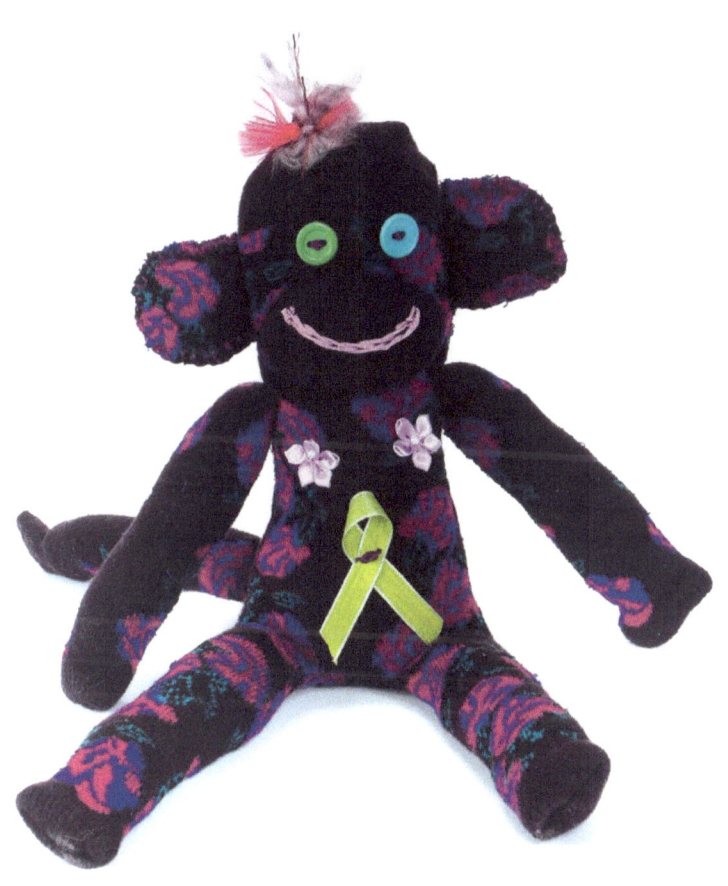

OLIVIA

Though her lustrous eyes and olive complexion gave Olivia a faintly exotic air, she was an unassuming sort. A long-time practitioner of mindfulness, her gentle demeanor was immediately felt by anyone in her sphere. Even her doctor fell under the influence of her calming, consoling ways. It was unsettling. Here he was doling out decidedly "bad" news, and Olivia merely gazed at him with her soothing expression. On the inside, Olivia saw her emotions twist and turn – sadness, fear, longing, resistance, anger and loss all played themselves out across the stage of her mind, but she knew that she was more than the sum of her feelings. There was a peaceful place, beyond the noisy fray of her mind and the roiling angst of her thoughts. She beckoned this stillness and watched it settle into her wide-open heart.

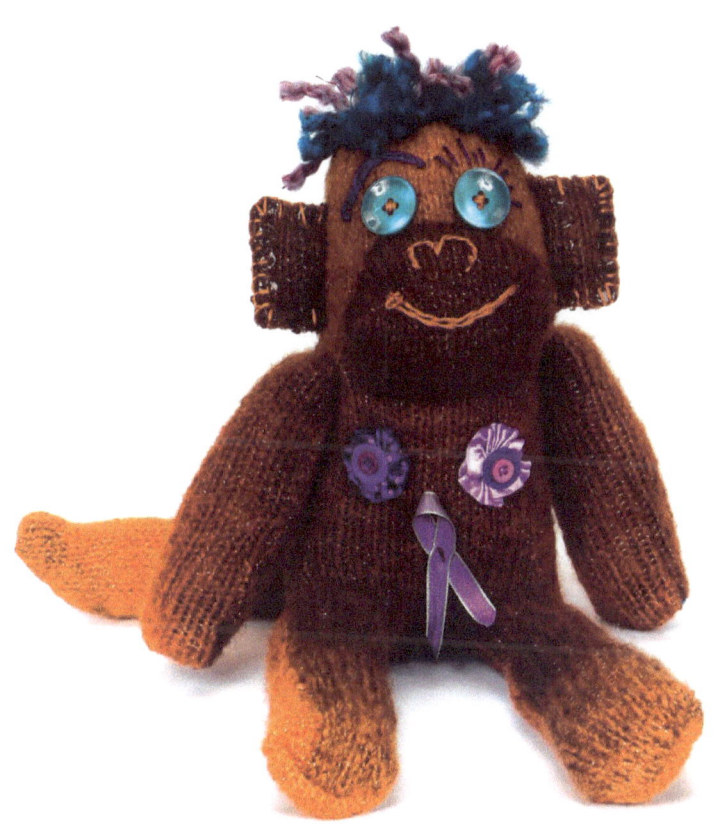

PEONY

Peony was baffled by the range of treatment options. In fact, she was completely overwhelmed. She had just exited the Oncologist's office, and she was more confused than ever. What was her next appropriate move? And what the hell had the Doctor just said? "Everyone should have at least one other person to accompany them to these appointments," she mused. "An advocate! Or at least another set of ears." There was simply so much information, far too much to absorb, and all of it was foreign to her regular line of thinking. So far, she had consulted with the Oncologist, her breast surgeon, the reconstructionist, and the radiologist. They all spoke rapidly from their respective arenas of expertise, and each seemed to propose a slight variation in her recommended treatment plan. It felt like she was getting conflicting stories everywhere she turned. Should she sign up to be part of the new drug trials at the University? Should she go for straight removal and hope they got it all? What if she made the "wrong" selection? The sheer volume of choices and the vast potential for wrong turns loomed menacingly. She hoped she could get to sleep that night.

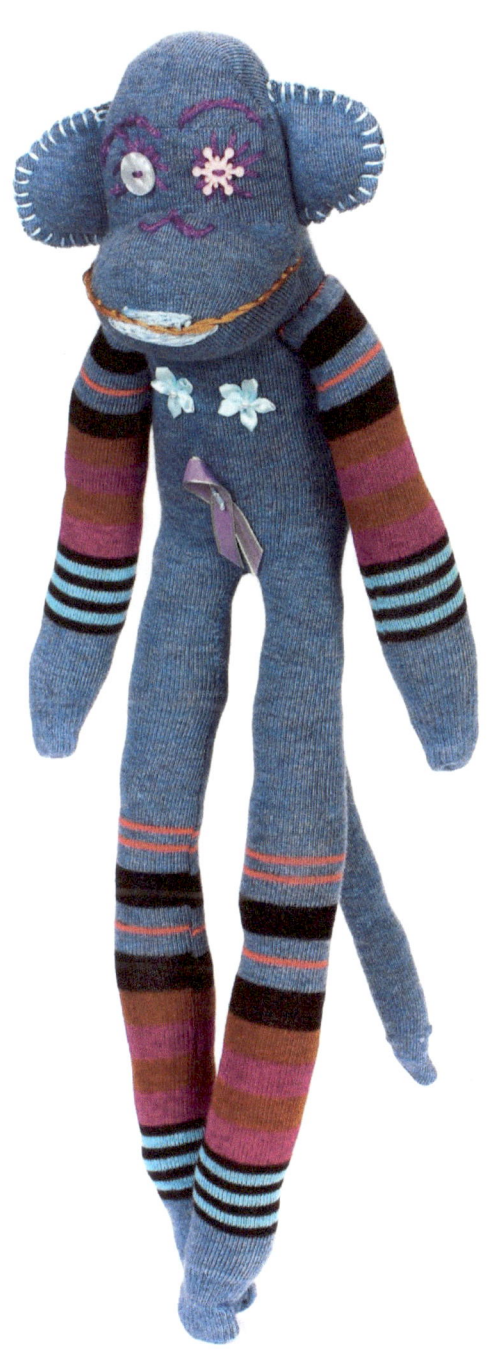

POSIE

Posie knew that all certainty was illusion, but what did that do to address her feelings, especially now that her sense of a "blankie" was ruthlessly stripped away. "Ignorance is bliss," or so the saying goes. And just now, Posie was feeling the full measure of that phrase. A deep processor at heart, Posie previously argued that such a state would hardly be bliss – for her at least. She was a meaning-maker from way back, and she longed to weave connections, and bring understanding to the most complex scenarios. But this breast cancer business was grinding her down, and, in her darkest moments, yes, she would say it...she craved ignorance! She wanted that cushiony sense of knowing that "everything would be okay." She longed to be enveloped by strong arms, with one hand stroking her head, and a gentle voice murmuring soft reassurances in her ear.

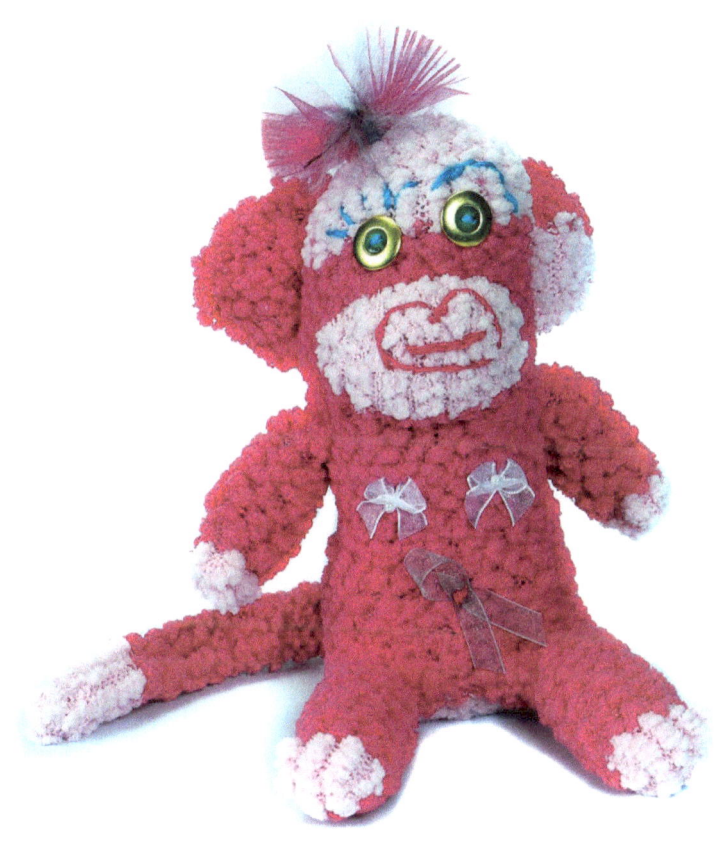

RUSTY

It was a definite curve ball. More than a bump in the road. Rusty wondered if it would end up being a "brick wall." Her family always said she was prone to making mountains out of mole hills. Did this qualify? Would a summer of radiation treatments really be "no big deal?" She didn't think so. Rusty pondered the way her family's judgments still ate at her, as though her parents would rush in at any moment to evaluate her actions. She knew they had good intentions. It's just that they wanted so badly to fix things and believed they had the corner market on the "correct" answers. Rusty thought life was less predictable yet somehow more meaningful than that, and she suspected there were some steep slopes ahead. She knew the coming months would challenge her perspective and that she would undoubtedly stumble repeatedly before finding her footing. "What if my 'mountain-making' has actually prepared me for this?" she mused.

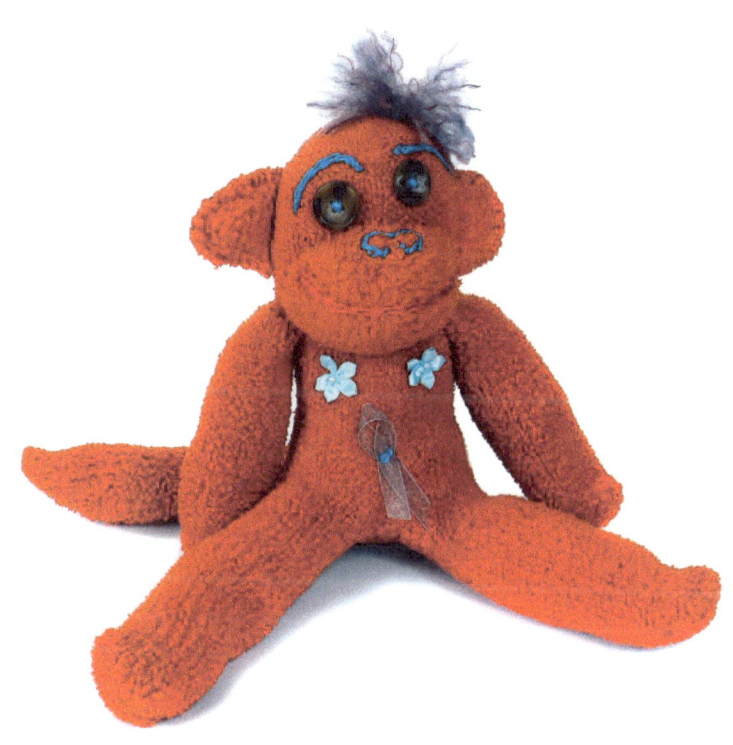

SUNSHINE

Sunshine veered out of orbit when news of her cancer came in. Her universe rapidly imploded and a stream of unleashed emotional fragments collided in a torrent around her. With the help of her family, friends, and colleagues, she slowly acclimated to the sinusoidal path as it unfolded, and her formerly rigid ways softened to embrace flexibility and change.

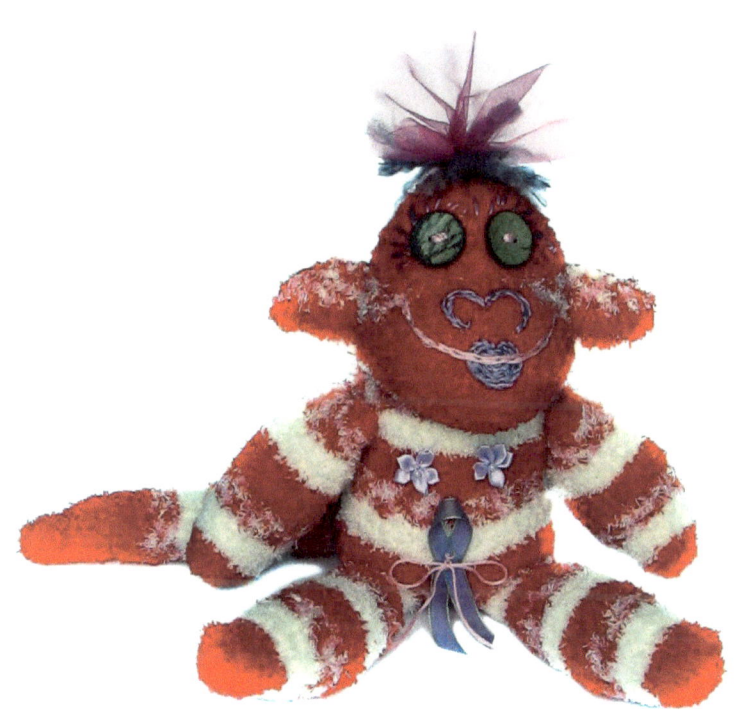

TOOTSIE

Tootsie's entire life revolved around sweetness. Her light and sugary presence added gaiety to every affair. She was like a puff of cotton candy. People even swore the scent of syrup wafted by whenever she passed. Long accustomed to such endearments as "Doll Face," "Pooh Bear," and "Cutie Pie," she was thrown completely off course by the words "breast cancer." Her? Really! She had never done anything wrong. She was entirely certain of it! She had done nothing to attract such an evil! She was so aggrieved, and so fierce in her denial, that she failed to notice that her friend, who normally only smiled in her presence, was staring at her in dismay. "Oh, Pooh Bear," he said, "don't you know that you didn't get breast cancer because you were bad? You just...simply...got it. It happens sometimes."

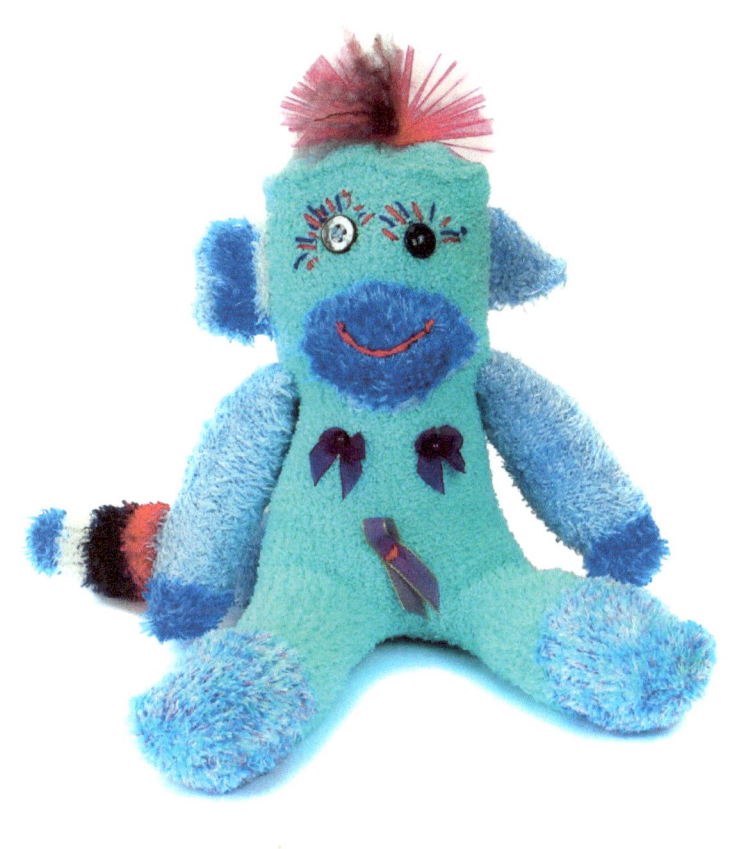

URSULA

The first-of-her-kind bear monkey, Ursula was
staggered by the force of the news. A young
mother with brand new cubs, she had eagerly
anticipated the swelling familial life ahead of her –
gorging on mountain blueberries, relishing the
gluttonous bounty of spawning season, and
nesting together at the onset of winter. The idea
that she had breast cancer was simply beyond
comprehension. She had life-saving instructions to
impart to her young; she had nourishment, love,
and wisdom to instill in their pliant youthful
hearts. "Well," she roared. She wasn't a bear
monkey for nothing! If ever she needed to call on
her genetic prowess and the favors of her
ancestral spirits, now was the time. It might
require a sheer force of will on her part, but she
was determined to find a life-giving route along
the precipitous path. She would find a way to bear
it, come what may.

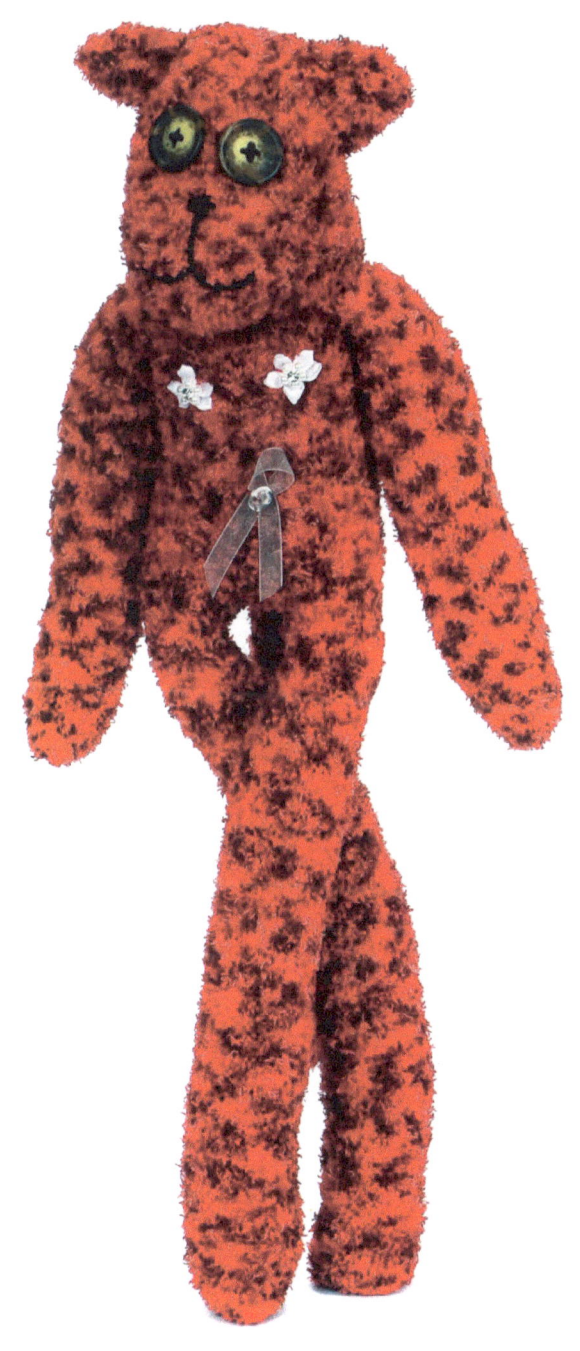

THE MONKEY STORY

"Oh, Sally..." she said, on opening it. For her 89th birthday, I had been sorely challenged to find anything...anything at all to breathe life into her spirit and make her days less long. But my mother's very first sock monkey surprised us both. Tears of delight blanketed her face. She stretched out her arms, reached for it, and simply stared. Her mouth curled gleefully into a little-girl smile, and with eyes glistening, she cooed again, "Oh, ohhhhh, Sally..."

Amazingly, the monkey conveyed my mother straight to her youth, offering a direct portal into carefree days, where "hope" colored her entire horizon.

"Miss Princess Annabelle Liberty Shores," aka "Gertrude," became my mother's new best friend. Mom proudly carted her along everywhere, and promptly enlisted the nurses, aides, and residents in a naming contest. To my sister and me, the monkey was unmistakably "Gertrude." But Mom insisted on her lengthier, more formal name. "Gertrude" became my mother's constant companion, and I quickly saw "more monkeys" move to the top of my to-do list.

"Gertrude" launched a four-month journey of unforeseen happiness, adding companionship, anticipation, and joy to each new day. Dozens of monkeys followed, and Mom hosted countless "sleep-overs" for her rapidly expanding group of friends. The new spark in Mom's eyes was never about me. It was the life force behind the monkeys themselves that formed the real gift. This new cast of characters carved out their own stories, each sending a taproot into Mom's most fanciful dreams and memories.

Mom's sock monkey journey was inexpressibly rich...a treasure trove of simple pleasures feeding her entire family. As she moved out of this life and into whatever follows, she cradled her friend, and I can only imagine she drew comfort from not passing alone.

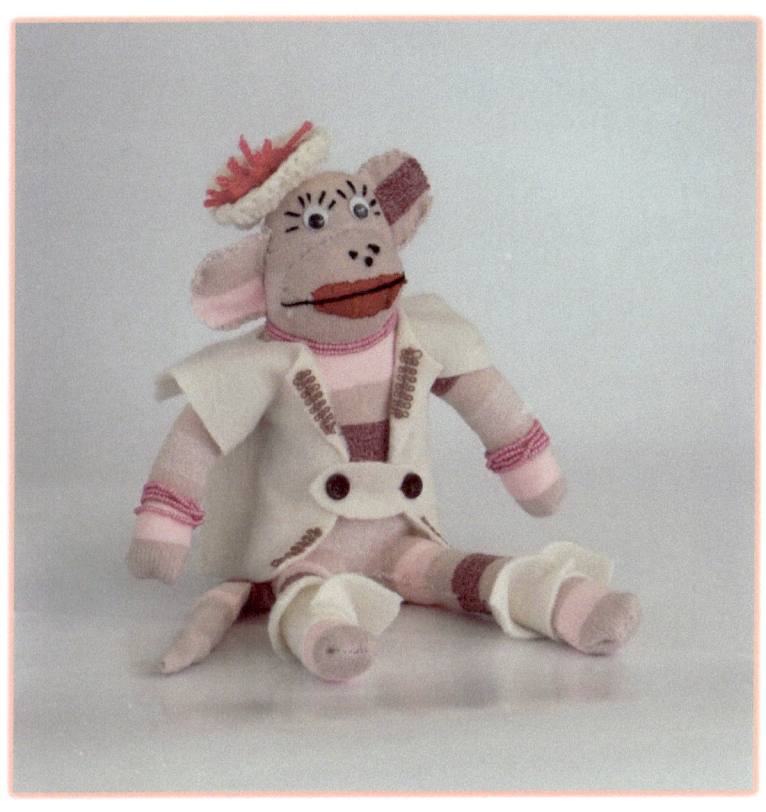

GERTRUDE

Gertrude's heavily-lashed eyes and wide red lips complement her somewhat misshapen limbs and strangely fashionable attire. The "original" monkey, she's undeniably ahead of her time and out of step with convention, but she's captivating in her ingenuity. Gertrude developed a special fascination for genealogy in her later years and recently discovered that she grew up a mere four miles from her contemporary, Agatha. Photo courtesy of Rex-zane Rudee.

ABOUT THE AUTHOR

Shaped by a free-range childhood in the Pacific Northwest, the author's work radiates from a deep and playful inner space.

As one among billions being human on the planet, she pairs language with design for clarity, beauty, and impact. Centering love as its compass, One Being Human gathers artistry, whimsy, and humility for each project.

Sally Jo's tiny 450sf home kindled her passion for minimalism and helped stretch her into the song she's here to sing. She's animated by peace, poetry, gardening, cooking, and sock monkeys.